I0423565

Disclaimer

Any application based on information in this book is at your own risk. The author is not liable for damages caused by applications due to the information contained in this book, and does **not give any promise of healing!**
It is recommended to consult a doctor.
The author has compiled the information with great conscience and care. No warranty is given for correctness. The author also accepts no liability for the content of linked Internet sites or other sources.

Foreword

Dear Reader,

my name is Christian.
I am glad that you have chosen my book.

Arteriosclerosis is still the number one cause of death in the Western industrial countries. To date, school medicine offers no satisfactory solutions. There are already a large number of scientific studies that have clearly demonstrated how vessel deposits can be solved. However, these studies apparently disappeared in the desk drawer and are so far only known in insider circles. As so often, only the public, which is also patentable and with which one can earn a lot of money. With my new immediate program against arteriosclerosis I show you (as always scientifically founded) how you can get back to clean blood vessels of a teenager.

Best regards,

Christian Meyer-Esch

You may also be interested in some of my other books:

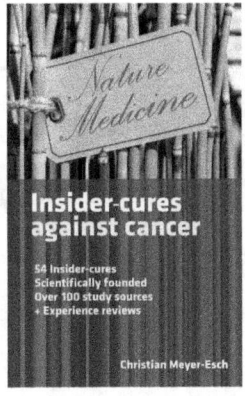

Insider-cures against cancer

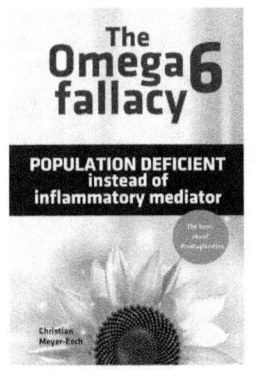

The Omega 6 fallacy: POPULATION DEFICIENT instead of inflammatory mediator

Contents

4

Atherosclerosis: What is it really?

Atherosclerosis ("hard arteries") is the common **"end product" of chronic inflammation:** deposits in the blood vessels, which ultimately lead to circulatory disorders. However, there are also vasoconstrictions and stiff blood vessels without deposits. You can also find out its causes in this book. However, these are not only calcium (lime) deposits. Also cholesterol, hardened connective tissue (fibrosis) and / or homocysteine narrow the arteries. Vascular deposition-induced arteriosclerosis is **always caused by chronic inflammation** *(study 6)*. You will find out how these inflammations come about and what this is all about, on the following pages.

How to diagnose atherosclerosis?

Unfortunately, there are only a few ways to diagnose atherosclerosis:

- Through an eye examination at the ophthalmologist (the retinal vessels of the eyes allow conclusions about the entire vascular situation of the body)

- The blood vessels can also be assessed by examining the carotid arteries by means of ultrasound **(carotid Doppler)**. From the nature of large arteries such as the throat lead, conclusions can be drawn about the blood flow situation, inter alia. Of heart and brain. However, what is difficult to diagnose are deposits in the fine capillary vessels. These are so tiny that only the blood corpuscles (blood cells) fit through. Even with the smallest deposits they are narrowed and can no longer do justice to their task. It is true that the body has the possibility of constantly forming new capillaries. However, is not sure how reliable this self-help measure is. Obviously not reliable enough, because otherwise there would be no heart attacks and strokes. At some point, finally, the end of the flagpole is reached. Of course you do not want that. You want to have lightning-clean blood vessels of a teenager and you should get this too.

What could happen if atherosclerosis remains untreated?

As you can imagine, untreated arteriosclerosis will continue to progress. Until some individual vessels are completely closed. Although the body reacts with self-help measures by forming new blood vessels and virtually creating the bypasses themselves. But that is not enough. This prevents the body from the worst, but the blood flow will still be worse than with healthy blood vessels.

The different forms of atherosclerosis

1. **Arterial calcification** (storage of calcium in the blood vessels)
2. **Fat deposits** (cholesterol, triglycerides and lipoprotein A)
3. **Homocysteine** (an amino acid that closes the vessels)
4. **Fibrosis** (Hardened collagen)
5. **Fibrin** (a clot-promoting adhesive protein)
6. **Arteriosclerosis without deposits** (a constriction of blood vessels when essential fatty acids or essential amino acids are deficient).

You can find out what the individual species mean on the following pages:

Blood vessels calcification

Calcium deposits are formed whenever two conditions are met:

1.) an inflammatory process must have preceded

2.) it there must be a deficiency of magnesium, inositol, lysine, vitamin D or vitamin K2.

On inflammation, the body reacts more frequently with the accumulation of calcium *(study 44)*. This, however, is not only in the blood vessels, but in principle everywhere. Above all, however, in tendons. These calcify very easily. Due to their testosterone, men are particularly susceptible to calcifications, because testosterone and their metabolites (dihydrotestosterone, DHT) promote calcification. **A study has shown that testosterone increases the calcification of blood vessels by 3 to 4 fold** *(study 43)*. This is probably the reason why men suffer a heart attack twice as often as women.

To clean blood vessels, it is, of course, now

our goal to dissolve these calcifications. For this purpose it is first of all important to eliminate the cause of the calcification: namely the chronic inflammation in the vessels! For information about these inflammations, see the chapter *"What causes the chronic inflammation of the arteries?"*

In addition there are 5 different means, which are able to solve the limescale deposits:
1. **Magnesium** (a mineral)
2. **Inositol** (a vitamin, namely the B8)
3. **Lysine** (an amino acid)
4. **Vitamin D** in the right dose (a hormone)
5. **Vitamin K2** (a vitamin)

But let us now go through the series of what the individual substances are and what they can:

Decalcification with Magnesium:

This mineral is known for muscle cramps. He is the opponent of calcium. It is estimated that a large part of the population has a deficiency of a magnesium and this leads to the fact that the calcium from the food or food supplements no longer reaches where it should go (ie into the bones and teeth), but in blood vessels, Tendons, and tissues, where of course there is nothing to look for. These limescale deposits then lead to so-called "stiffness" over the years. One can also imagine magnesium as a "plasticizer". Calcium makes hard, magnesium soft. And there must always be a balanced balance of two. We want hard teeth and bones, but also soft and elastic blood vessels. According to the German Society for Nutrition, the daily time for magnesium is 300-400 mg / day. Women need something less, men need something more. In scientific investigations it was found that magnesium taken orally leads to a recovery of limescale deposits in the whole body, also in the blood vessels *(studies 46, 47)*. Eighty patients with soft tissue laxation participated in a study. Magnesium was also administered orally, as well as locally. After 20 weeks, 75% of all patients were cured of limescale deposits. However, magnesium can also be injected or become in the form of plasters. However, so-called penetration agents are needed in order to penetrate the active substances through the skin barrier, for example propylene glycol (a special alcohol is available in every pharmacy). Still more tolerant is dimethyl sulfoxide (DMSO) or organic sulfur (MSM).

The highest magnesium contents are on 100 grams: cocoa powder (about 400 mg), dark chocolate (about 300 mg), cashews (about 250 mg), soy products and almonds (approx. 250 mg), peanuts (about 160 mg), Wholemeal bread (about 150 mg), oat flakes (about 140 mg), beans (about 130 mg), wholemeal flour (about 130 mg). Anyone suffering from circulatory disorders should also take magnesium as a supplement to meet the requirements of 400 mg. In my opinion, the recommendations of the US Society for Nutrition are much too low. Especially if limescale deposits already exist, so it already 1.000 mg / day be. Many are wondering which art of magnesium would be most suitable: magnesium citrate, magnesium carbonate, magnesium chloride or others. According to scientific studies, the best magnesium forms are magnesium citrate and magnesium gluconate. Very badly cut off the magnesium oxide. This is as good as not bioavailable. All other magnesium forms are somewhere in the middle. Are also relatively bio available. In the investigations, it was also found that the organic magnesium compounds are more bioavailable than inorganic. The difference is not only minimal *(studies 48, 49, 51, 52)*. The magnesium from the mineral water is also bioavailable *(Study 50)*.

Decalcification with Inositol (Vitamin B8):

It is probably next to B15 and B17 the most unknown B-vitamin. Unjustly, because inositol specifically engages in the hormonal balance and regulates it. Many hormone-related diseases such as PCOS syndrome, excessive body hair (especially in women), acne, premenstrual syndrome and much more have already been cured with inositol. But that is another issue. Here we are concerned with the lime-removing effect of the inositol, which so far is only known in insider circles.

Inositol is a hexavalent alcohol found in both plants and animals. This is present in the human body practically in all tissues. High concentrations are found in the brain, eyes, heart muscles, in the kidneys, liver and spleen as well as in the testes. Inositol can be produced by the body itself from glucose and is therefore considered non-essential. It may also be formed from healthy bacterial cultures in the digestive tract. Inositol is contained in the food mainly in oranges, nuts, beans, wheat and wheatgrass. It occurs in the form of phytic acid. If these are absorbed in large quantities from food, they can reduce the absorption of calcium, iron and zinc. Inositol from food supplements does not have this effect and is therefore the appropriate means for therapeutic purposes. Although inositol carries the trivial name "muscle sugar", it is not a carbohydrate because it has no carbonyl group. It only fulfills the original criterion of a carbohydrate (hydrated carbon). This close relative of choline (vitamin B4) and biotin (vitamin B7) works closely together with vitamin B6, folic acid (vitamin B9) and pantothenic acid (vitamin B5) and is a component of lecithin. It protects liver, kidneys, heart and veins. Very high coffee consumption can empty the inositol stores in the body. Inositol is a distinct brain food. It plays a role in human metabolism as myo-inositol, its content is quite high in the organs. In animal experiments, inositol repaired neural tube defects and high doses showed marked antidepressant effects, while an inositol deficiency led to liver fatting. To produce this substance itself, the body needs abundant niacin (vitamin B3) and magnesium. Above all, the latter is lackware. Even in alternative medical circles, the fact that inositol is also able to bring lime (calcium) to where it belongs is in the bones and teeth and thus removed from the blood vessels. Several studies *(58, 59, 60, 61)* demonstrated that inositol inhibits calcification. In one study, e.g. Rat calcium administered with a concurrent diet low in inositol. These rats were found to have calcifications of the coronary vessels, whereas in rats whose diet was rich in inositol, calcification did not occur *(Study 58)*. A further study *(68)* also showed that an inositol cream is also capable of dissolving local calcium deposits in the skin. It was also found in these rats that the inositol was detected in the urine. This indicates that the external inositol application is well bioavailable and enters the bloodstream. Important: Insoitol should always be taken with vitamin B5 (pantothenic acid), otherwise it can not be absorbed by the body or can not be adequately absorbed *(study 57)*.

Decalcification with Lysine:

Also hardly known as lime inhibitors is the amino acid lysine *(study 62)*. Lysine is one of the 8 essential amino acids that the body can not produce by itself and therefore has to be fed with the food. Lysine ensures that the calcium is removed from the blood vessels and gets into the teeth and bones. Lysine-rich foods are Parmesan, soybeans, wheat germs, lentils, peanuts (among others). Of course there is also lysine as a dietary supplement kiloweise as a powder to buy. The daily requirement is approximately 15 mg / kg (milligram per kilogram of body weight). That is, a 70 kg human being, for example, needs 1050 mg a day.

Decalcification with Vitamin D:

For this, one must first say: **ONLY in the right dose!** Because both too little and too much Vitamin D leads to calcification. Only the right amount works against calcification! Vitamin D is mainly known as so-called "sun-vitamin", because it is formed by solar radiation in the organism. The term "vitamin" has become so natural, but actually vitamin D is not a vitamin, but a hormone. The term "vitamin D" refers to a group of fat-soluble compounds which are used as pre-hormones or hormone precursors. The active form of vitamin D is called calcitriol. Among the well-known forms of vitamin D is vitamin D3 (cholecalciferol), which is synthesized from the sun in the skin. The initial form of vitamin D (7-dehydrocholesterol) travels to the liver, where it is converted to another more active form of vitamin D, the 25-hydroxyvitamin D (calcifediol). This is the vitamin D form, which also examines laboratories for deficiencies in the blood. When vitamin D leaves the liver, it travels to the kidneys where it is once again converted into the highly metabolically active form of vitamin D called calcitriol or 1,25 dihydroxyvitamin D. This is no more than vitamin, but steroid hormone. Calcitriol increases calcium absorption from food in our digestive tract. Here again step by step from sun exposure in the skin to the active vitamin D:

1. **7-Dehydrocholesterol**

   (Shot through the skin in the sun)
2. **Cholecalciferol**
3. Transformation in the liver to:
4. **25-Hydroxyvitamin D3**
5. Transformation in the kidneys to:
6. **1,25 Dihydroxyvitamin D3**

The daily requirement of vitamin D is about 200-600 international units (IU). **The skin produces approximately 10,000 IU of vitamin D after total irradiation with UV light** *(study 63)*. The currently tolerable intake in Europe and North America is 50 micrograms / day (2000 IU / day). Clinical studies show that a longer intake of 10,000 IU is probably not a risk *(study 63)*. Doses of more than 50,000 IU / day increase the values of 25 (OH) vitamin D to more than 150 ng / ml and are associated with hypercalcemia and hyperphosphatemia **(risk of arteriosclerosis)!** From what daily dose of vitamin D an overdose occurs, is not yet scientifically clarified. The current recommendations are 2,000 IU per day. It is best to combine vitamin D with magnesium, lysine, inositol and vitamin K2, so that the calcium can also get into the bones and teeth and does not settle in the blood vessels.

The optimal blood value of vitamin D is 35-60 nanograms per milliliter or 80-150 nanomoll per liter.

Decalcification with Vitamin K2:

There are 3 types of vitamin K:
K1 (Phylloquinone) = mainly found in green leafy vegetables and is mainly known for its anticoagulant properties. In the organism it is stored in liver, kidney, bone marrow and spleen.
K2 (menaquinone) = has *decalcification* properties on the blood vessels. This form is interesting for us!

K3 = is a <u>non</u>-recommended synthetic vitamin K.

The vitamin K-dependent protein, matrix GLA protein (MGP), is a central calcification inhibitor produced by the vascular smooth muscle cells and regulates the potentially lethal accumulation of calcium in the blood vessels. In contrast to vitamin K1 (which occurs in green plants), vitamin K2 is produced by bacteria of the intestinal flora when vitamin K1 is sufficiently present. Vitamin K1 intake in children has declined significantly since 1950 *(study 64)*. Vitamin K2 has shown profound effects on the reduction of blood vessel calcification. It was noted that the arterial calcification of cultured bovine aortic gland muscle cells treated with inorganic phosphate was reduced. In another study, vitamin K2 reduced the progress of arteriosclerosis in hypercholesteroleic rabbits. In addition, vitamin K2 can improve the lipid profile by increasing HDL levels and lowering overall cholesterol levels. Recognizing the effect of vitamin K2 on reducing the risk of coronary heart disease, the International Life Sciences Institute (ILSI

Europe) recommends the use of vitamin K2 in addition to K1. While vitamin K2 is being studied for its role in the modulation of calcification, K1 appears to have no significant effect on vascular calcification, as has been shown in several studies. Vitamin K antagonists such as warfarin and its derivatives, are administered as anticoagulants to many patients. They have been found to cause calcification in human thigh arteries, mitral valves, aortic valves, carotid artery, and aorta. According to a meta-analysis, the risk of myocardial infarction or stroke is significantly increased when calcium supplements are taken. In the case of calcium-rich diet, however, no increased risk was found *(study **65**)*. Important epidemiological evidence has shown that the serum calcium in the upper part of the normal range is a risk factor for vascular diseases and that calcium preparations raise the serum calcium acutely. In a study in rats it was shown that vitamin K2 was able to reduce the calcium deposits in the blood vessels by 50%. *(Study **66**)*.

Rich in K2 is the Japanese specialty "Natto". From which the K2 in capsule form is also won. For the production, soybeans are boiled and subsequently fermented by the action of the bacterium Bacillus subtilis natto. An increased intake of menachinone (vitamin K2) was also associated with a **35% reduction in cancer risk**. But this is only by the way. You can find out more about in my book *"Insider-cures against cancer"*. (www.insider-remedies.com)

Tip: Vitamin K2 as MK-7: There are different forms of vitamin K2! But only the MK-7 has a half-life of 2.5 days. This means that after 2.5 days the vitamin is reduced by half. With other K2 forms one has a complete dismantling already after few hours! Only the MK-7 thus provides a 24-hour care without having to swallow a tablet every 3 hours.

Fat deposits (lipoprotein A, cholesterol and triglycerides)

Lipoprotein A:

This parameter is usually (like all values, which are really important) not taken over by the statutory health insurance funds. After all, you can only earn money with sick people.

Normal value of lipoprotein A in blood serum:
Up to 30 mg / dl. (Milligrams per deciliter)
or
Up to 75 nmol / l (nanomoll per liter)

Lipoprotein A is a low density lipoprotein (LDL) containing the protein chains "Apolipoprotein A1" and "Apolipoprotein B 100". In particular, the length of this chain depends on whether the lipoprotein A value in the blood is high or low. Some diseases may lead to an increased lipoprotein A value secondary:

- *Kidney disease*
- *Diabetes*
- *Thyroid function under (hypothyroidism)*

You can imagine the lipoprotein A as an adhesive. It is LDL cholesterol + adhesive. And this combination is, of course, very unfavorable, since it closes the vessels. Too high lipoprotein A levels prevent plasminogen from forming the blood clot-dissolving plasmin and thus microthrombi can not be resolved. If these become detached from the vessel wall, a life-threatening embolism, a heart attack or a stroke can occur. Therefore, it is important to keep the lipoprotein A level low so that blood clots can be made liquid and therefore can not lead to vessel closure. If you have an elevated lipoprotein A level in your blood, a deficiency of vitamin C, lysine, niacin (vitamin B3) as well as L-carnitine can be behind it. As a result, the lipoprotein A level decreases when the above-mentioned vital substances are again available in an adequate amount. Unfortunately, there are hereditary elevated mirrors, which can not be reduced by absorbing the above-mentioned vital substances. In such a case, mental healing (quantum healing) might be a therapy option. Normal naturopathy will not work in such a case unfortunately, or the Wunderkraut was not yet found. This book is mainly about the elevated lipoprotein A-levels caused by living circumstances and not the hereditary. The question is, of course, why does the body produce lipoprotein A at all, if it is so harmful to the vessels? Does our organism want to destroy itself? No. Rather, lipoprotein A serves as a kind of "flicker tool". If you have leaking blood vessels, for example because of a vitamin C deficiency, then the body tries to stick these fine cracks: Using lipoprotein A! The only problem is that when these deposits get the upper hand somehow the corresponding vessel is eventually completely closed. If the body did not have lipoprotein A then the vessels would not be able to be patched again and we would bleed to death. And although elevated lipoprotein A levels are associated with arteriosclerosis, there is so far no evidence that a decrease in elevated values reduces the risk of cardiovascular disease *(study 53)*. Nevertheless, it must be noted that healthy people do not have elevated lipoprotein A levels and therefore a reduction seems necessary for the cause.

And so simply lower the lipoprotein A level with natural vital substances:

Reduction of lipoprotein A by niacin (vitamin B3):

Studies showed a decrease of lipoprotein A dose-dependent by a maximum of 30-40%. In the case of niacin, you should ensure that it is pure nicotinic acid, which also has the so-called "flush effect". This means that the blood vessels are taken after the niacin intake for c. 30-60 minutes greatly expanded. There is heat, sweating and itching. Afterwards, one becomes very cold and tired. You should therefore take Niacin in the evening before going to bed. Make sure that it is not the niacinamide. So whenever amid is at the end, it is niacin with no flushing effect and you should not buy it, as the flush is just as important to detoxify the body. The dosage should be at least 500 mg / day. Usually 500 mg for an optimal flush effect. However, be careful not to buy niacin with delayed delivery, as these are suspected to damage the liver. In addition to lipoprotein A, niacin also lowers LDL cholesterol and triglycerides *(study 954)*.

Reduction of lipoprotein A by Vitamin C:

Surely you've heard a lot about the seasickness scurvy. This is triggered by a chronic vitamin C deficiency for months: The sailors bled to death. Vitamin C ensures that the blood vessel walls remain clean and elastic. In the absence of vitamin C or even in the complete lack of vitamin C in the diet, the blood vessels become perforated and porous. In this case, the lipoprotein A is used to repair the defective blood vessels. Experiments in mice showed that the lipoprotein A level is parallel to vitamin C uptake. When the vitamin C intake was sufficiently high, lipoprotein A levels *(study 54)* decreased. Take at least 1 g (1,000 mg) of vitamin C per day. Ideally combined with a juice. For example, Drink orange juice and dissolve in these pure ascorbic acid, then it is significantly healthier than if you consume the vitamin C pure (without juice). One study showed that vitamin C-rich orange juice reduced DNA damage by free oxygen radicals by 18%. The water with pure vitamin C did not happen. Vitamin C acts when it is taken up pure, not anti-but pro-oxidative! This means it becomes a free radical itself. Only in combination with other vitamins and secondary plantings does it unfold its antioxidant effect and protects the organism including the blood vessels from damage *(study 855)*.

Reduction of lipoprotein A by L-carnitine:

L-carnitine: What is it actually? This is a chemical compound, which is produced from the amino acids lysine and methionine. It plays a decisive role in energy metabolism as well as in the transport of fatty acids. The body can independently produce L-carnitine when the following "ingredients" are present:

- *Lysine*
- *Methionine*
- *Vitamin C*
- *Vitamin B6*
- *Iron*
- *Niacin (Vitamin B3)*

In studies, L-carnitine has been shown to be

able to significantly reduce elevated lipoprotein A levels *(Studies 55, 56)*.

Reduction of lipoprotein A by L-Lysine:

The essential amino acid lysine you know already as a means against limescale deposits in the vessels. However, it is also significantly involved in collagen formation. It also ensures that the collagen-releasing enzymes are inhibited, so that the blood vessels remain clean and elastic. In addition, together with vitamin C and the non-essential amino acid proline, it forms a kind of Teflon layer in the vessels and ensures that both lipoprotein A is degraded and no further lipoprotein A can adhere to the vessels. And this is above all not symptomatic, but because it is no longer needed because of the lysine. The dose should be 5-10 g per day.

Cholesterol:

Surely, your doctor has often already measured the cholesterol level. Besides the total cholesterol level there is the LDL cholesterol (so-called "bad" cholesterol) and the HDL (so-called "good" cholesterol). Therefore, LDL cholesterol is most relevant to health. Because cholesterol was found after heart attacks in the plaques of the vascular walls, it was thought that reducing this substance had beneficial effects. But there is still no study that could prove that cholesterol is the cause of atherosclerosis. Cholesterol-rich foods hardly affect cholesterol levels. *(Study 8)*. Because the body produces and regulates the cholesterol level itself. If a lot of cholesterol is needed, the body produces a lot of cholesterol. If he needs less, his own production is throttled. If, therefore, a lot of cholesterol is already consumed by the diet, the body restricts the body's production. Cholesterol: What exactly is it? This is a waxy mass, precisely a polycyclic alcohol, which practically every body organism desperately needs. And because this waxy mass can not float freely in the blood, it is bound to transport proteins:

HDL = high density lipoprotein: Supposedly "good" cholesterol. (High density lipoprotein) is transported back to the liver by the body organs.

LDL = low density lipoprotein: Supposedly "bad" cholesterol (Low-density lipoprotein) is transported from the liver into the bloodstream to all possible organs.

And then there is: **VLDL = Very Low Density Lipoprotein:** With this lipoprotein, triglycerides, phospholipids and cholesterol are mainly transported from the liver to the body's circulation. More than 90 percent of the cholesterol is produced in the liver. Previously it was thought that a high cholesterol level was due to the dietary intake. But today it is known that this is not so. The pharmaceutical industry has, however, discovered a brilliant billions of business through the cholesterol buyers (so-called "statins"). The standard value of the cholesterol level in the laboratory has been steadily declining and the business of anxiety has continued to grow. But let's look at what cholesterol is so important:

1.) Construction of the cell membrane

One of the most important tasks of cholesterol is to stabilize the cell membrane. Each cell is surrounded by a cell membrane. A cell always builds more cholesterol into the membrane when toxins are present in the environment (which we also call a matrix). These can come through the food, be produced by vaccinations or by metabolic products themselves. Any inflammation is a danger to the body cell and thus increases the cholesterol level. Chronic inflammation, in particular, greatly increases the cholesterol level. The body thus has an intelligent self-regulation.

2.) Building blocks for the hormones

A sufficient amount of cholesterol is necessary to build up and maintain the hormone balance. Our stress hormone cortisone and also the sex hormones need the building block cholesterol. A deficiency therefore leads to a hormonal subfunction. Also the "sun vitamin" D3, actually also a hormone, consists mainly of cholesterol. It is responsible for the metabolism, the immune system and the bone structure. A deficiency of vitamin D3 leads to osteoporosis. If the cholesterol sinker results in a reduced provision of this building block, the immune system, the hormones and the bone structure suffer. Also the cancer risk is increased by vitamin D3 deficiency. More in my book *"Insider-cures against cancer"*. In the case of arteriosclerosis, both a vitamin D level that is too low and too high a vitamin D level results in calcium deposits in the vessels.

3.) Cholesterol for the brain and nervous system

Most cholesterol is found in the brain. Cholesterol is one of the factors that causes nerve cells (neurons) to come into contact and exchange electrical signals. Cholesterol is formed by glial cells, which form a large part of the brain tissue and support its development and function in a variety of ways. The function of the nervous system is based on the exchange of electrical signals between nerve cells, which is mediated via highly specialized contact points, so-called synapses.

But where does the myth come from, cholesterol would lead to deposits in the vessels? It has probably begun with a few innocent rabbits who had to deal with studies of arteriosclerosis and cholesterol. The rabbits were fed cholesterol until their vessels slowly began to accumulate. This experiment is regarded as ancestor of the theory: Cholesterol consumption is unhealthy, cholesterol leads to arteriosclerosis. But rabbits are vegetarians and in their typical diet no cholesterol occurs at all. The natural cholesterol value of rabbits is about 45 mg / dl. However, the rabbits were so heavily fed until their levels increased to about 1200 mg / dl, which is equivalent to poisoning of the animals. This corresponds to a cholesterol level of approximately 7,000 mg / dl.

Now, however, there are people whose cholesterol levels are low and those with high cholesterol levels. So the question is: 1.) a high cholesterol level is bad and 2.) why do some people have so much cholesterol in the blood? To answer the first question: yes and no. A high cholesterol level is bad in so far as it indicates that something is not quite right with the body at the moment. However, it would be even worse if the body was something wrong and the cholesterol level would not be increased. You need to imagine cholesterol as a kind of "fire service". Whenever the body needs to repair a lot, cholesterol levels rise. For example, if you are hurt and a lot of nerve cells have been affected, it is quite normal that the cholesterol level rises to repair the broken nerve cells. The same also with blood vessels: If these are chronically inflamed and microscopically small cracks form, the body reacts with the distribution of cholesterol, in order to seal the vessel damage. Therefore, it makes no sense to swallow statins (cholesterol-lowering drugs). For these only suppress the symptom. It would be different if the statins themselves were able to repair the vessel damage and the cholesterol would simply not be needed. But that is not the case. Thus, the body is not pleased to quasi suppress the body-borne fire service. That would be fatal. And why some people have an increased cholesterol level, you know now as well. In the body is something broken, which must be repaired or patched. The goal must therefore be to reduce the cholesterol level to a healthy level, but not by statins, but in which the body itself says "I do not need many cholesterol anymore". Therefore, e.g. Also lecithin is a very good means to lower cholesterol levels. The nerve cells are surrounded by a myelin layer. This is where lecithin comes in and provides new materials for the scaffolding of nerve cells. Lecithin is a mixture of choline (vitamin B4), inositol (vitamin B8) and phospholipids. Just the right building material for nerve cells. As a result, the cholesterol level decreases all the time because cholesterol is no longer needed. Niacin (vitamin B3) is also able to significantly reduce cholesterol levels. The risk of myocardial infarction could not be reduced *(studies **67**, **68**)*.

<u>Normal value for LDL cholesterol:</u>
Very low: below 70 mg / dl
Low: 70-100 mg / dl
Normal: 100-130 mg / dl
High limit: 130-160 mg / dl
High: 160-190 mg / dl
Very high: 190 mg and above

<u>Normal value for HDL cholesterol:</u>
At least 45 mg / dl (the higher the better!)

<u>Normal value for total cholesterol:</u>
Up to 200 mg / dl (the lower the better!)

Triglycerides

Triglycerides are so-called neutral fats. They are absorbed both by food and by the liver itself. The body stores triglycerides in adipose tissue and releases them with increased energy requirements. In 3. world countries, the triglyceride level is often increased. Nevertheless, these people rarely develop a cardiovascular disease such as myocardial infarction *(study 31)*. Other studies have found a link between myocardial infarction and elevated triglyceride levels, while others do not. The scientific study situation is very spongy. Concrete evidence is missing. Since high triglyceride levels are often observed in patients with metabolic syndrome and type 2 diabetes (study 31-2), these diseases could be responsible for the increased risk of myocardial infarction than the triglycerides themselves To reduce the triglyceride level is lecithin. This is a mixture of choline (vitamin B4), inositol (vitamin B8) and phospholipids. This is available as granules in drugstore stores cheap. Of course, I can not make any promises of healing, but so many people have already reduced their triglyceride levels. Niacin (vitamin B3) is also able to lower triglyceride levels. In addition, niacin also inhibits inflammation and oxidative stress, and that is precisely the reason for arteriosclerosis *(study 31-3)*.

Normal value for triglycerides:
Up to 200 mg / dl (the lower the better!)

Homocysteine

Homocysteine is a naturally occurring, non-proteinogenic α-amino acid. It is an intermediate in human amino acid metabolism, more specifically in the degradation of methionine (also an amino acid). This amino acid has to be fed daily over the food and serves the body u.a. As an important sulfur source. Homocysteine, on the other hand, is a poisonous waste product and is therefore quickly bound, converted back into methionine by means of vitamin B9 and B12 or further degraded with the help of vitamin B6 and excreted mostly through the kidneys.

Homocysteine is therefore unhealthy because it causes inflammation in the blood vessels and so over the years calcium, cholesterol, and fibrin deposits are formed in the blood vessels that occlude them. Through the enjoyment of coffee, alcohol, cigarettes as well as overweight and lack of exercise, increased homocysteine values occur. **But above all, when there is a lack of the B vitamins B6, B9 and B12 and Lecithine**.

Methionine (present in meat, fish, and cheese) is metabolised by the vitamin B6-dependent reaction. As laboratory markers, the level of homocysteine level after methionine administration is considered as a test for possible genetic defects. Also a vitamin B6 deficiency causes a homocysteine increase after a methionine-rich diet. In medicine, **a homocysteine level of up to 5 micromol / liter is ideal.** However, since this value can hardly be adjusted in older people, a homocysteine level of up to 8 micromol / liter is still classified as inconspicuous in most cases *(source 2)*. But also my older readers are not satisfied with values of 8 of course. They do not want "acceptable" values, but ideal values of a teenager.

Homocysteine value up to 5: "Too low" does not exist with homocysteine

= Dream value! Only this we should accept and strive for. Do not settle for less! How many people among the lucky with such values are, is not known. It should be less than 5%.

Homocysteine value 6 to 8: "Good but not good enough"

= Have only 10% of the European population. Such values are considered as healthy, but from my point of view not as optimal.

Homocysteine value from 9 to 11: Below average risk

35% of the European population lives with this value.

Homocysteine value of 12 to 14: Average risk

20% of the European population lives with this value

Homocysteine value of 15 to 17: Risk slightly increased

Health is already suffering, even if no symptoms have developed. 20% of the European population belong to this category.

Homocysteine value from 18 to 19: High risk

This category has a high risk with a 50% chance of developing a stroke, heart attack, cancer or Alzheimer within the next 10 to 30 years. 10% of the European population lives with these very high values.

Homocysteine value of 20 and above: Highest risk

These are peak values with the extremely high risk of being haunted by one of the five major civilization diseases: heart attack, stroke, diabetes, cancer, dementia. 5% of the European population lives in this highest risk area.

Distribution of homocysteine levels in the population:

Only 10% of the population lives with optimal homocysteine values:

Hcy value <8: 10%

Homocysteine value <12: 35%

Homocysteine value <15: 20%

Homocysteine value <18: 20%

Homocysteine value <20: 10%

Homocysteine value> 20: 5%

Any increase in 5 micromoles / liter of homocysteine in the blood increases the risk of cardiovascular events by about 20%, regardless of conventional risk factors such as e.g. Smoking or diabetes (*study* **69**).

Fibrosis (Hardened connective tissue)

Fibrosis is called hard, thick connective tissue. This is defined by the overgrowth, hardening and / or scarring of various tissues. Fibrosis is the end result of chronic inflammatory responses induced by a variety of stimuli, including infections, autoimmune responses, allergic reactions, toxins, radiation, and tissue injury. The problem with fibrosis is that it makes the blood vessels hard and impermeable. Fibrosis of the blood vessels can not be diagnosed. It is indisputable, however, that fibrosis occurs in arteriosclerosis *(study 42)*. Not causing, but at least significantly promoting, the male sex hormones testosterone as well as its degradation product (the dihydrotestosterone, also called DHT) do the fibrosis *(study 42-2)*. Men therefore have significantly more fibrosis than women and children. Probably also with the main reason why men are more likely to suffer from arteriosclerosis than women. Fibrosis, however, affects not only chronically inflamed blood vessels, but also the heart tissue *(study 42-3)*. It has important consequences for heart function and leads to increased mechanical stiffness and diastolic dysfunction. In addition, the fibrosis can interfere with an electrical coupling, resulting in impaired cardiac contraction. In addition, inflammation and fibrosis in the perivascular (near a vessel) areas can reduce the flow of oxygen and nutrients and increase the pathological remodeling (bone remodeling). What means help to resolve fibrosis? According to current knowledge, there are only a few remedies for fibrosis, namely Mariendistel *(study 42-4)*, the B3 vitamin niacin *(study 42-5)* and the amino acid degradation product taurine *(study 42-6)*. This is produced in the metabolism as a degradation product of the amino acids cysteine and methionine, but can also be purchased as a dietary supplement in tablet or powder form. The Mariendistel has long been known as a remedy for liver diseases. Also, the liver can develop a fibrosis and studies showed that the Mariendistel was able to break down these. Although there are no explicit studies on the presence of fibrosis on the heart or the blood vessels, the Mariendistel is not only effective against fibrosis in the liver, but also against fibrosis in all parts of the body. It must be said that the topic of fibrosis is relatively new in medicine. Large-scale studies are missing and so we must be satisfied with the means by which the probability of the fibrosis dissolving is high.

Fibrinogen and Fibrin

The extent to which vessels are contaminated with fibrin deposits can not be diagnosed. It is indisputable, however, that these fibrin deposits occur *(studies **38**, **39**)*. The blood clotting factor I (fibrinogen), is a glycoprotein (macromolecule consisting of protein and bound carbohydrates), which is formed in the liver. Coagulation factors are substances which, in the event of an injury, ensure that the blood coagulates and thus the bleeding can be stopped. The body then converts fibrinogen to fibrin. Imagine fibrin as a cobweb-like scaffold that closes the bleeding wound. Elevated fibrinogen levels may indicate inflammation in the body and are a risk factor for atherosclerosis. In advanced plaque, fibrin can be involved in the tight binding of LDL. Thus, there is extensive evidence that increased blood coagulation is a risk factor not only for thrombotic occlusion, but also for atherosclerosis. Higher blood coagulation often coexists with hyperlipidemia (high cholesterol / lipoprotein A) and together these can have a synergistic effect on arteriosclerosis. The standard value for fibrinogen is 1.5 - 4.0 g / l for adults. As already mentioned, it is unfortunately not possible to determine the extent to which the vessels already exhibit fibrin deposits. Let us assume that these fibrin deposits are present.

How can we dissolve the fibrin deposits without injuring the blood vessel? By the enzyme of silkworms: **Serrapeptase**. In contrast to cholesterol-lowering drugs (statins), **the serrapeptase clears the fibrin deposits from the arterial wall without affecting cholesterol synthesis.** The enzyme serrapeptase has fibrin-dissolving properties: it is easily digested! It has been used for over 20 years, is available as an over-the-counter dietary supplement and no known side effects are known to date. Large-scale studies, especially with regard to arteriosclerosis, are missing. However, its fibrin-dissolving effect is clearly demonstrated in studies. For example, a double-blind, placebo-controlled study was conducted to investigate the clinical efficacy of serrapeptase in a total of 174 patients. 88 patients received 10 mg serrapeptase 3 times the day before surgery, once in the night of surgery and 3 times daily for 5 days after surgery. The other 86 patients received a placebo. The degree of swelling in patients treated with serrapeptase was significantly lower than in the placebo-treated patients until the 5th day. No adverse reactions were reported *(study 71)*.

Dosage suggestion: 80,000 IU or IU (international units) per day. Make sure the tablets are designed to be resistant to gastric juice! Otherwise, the tablet would already dissolve in the stomach and thus would be ineffective!

Atherosclerosis without vascular deposits

Also independent of deposits in the blood vessels can cause bleeding disturbances! This is due to vasoconstriction. Triggered by:

- **Deficient of the amino acids L-Arginine and L-Citrulline**
- **Deficient of prostaglandins (tissue hormones)**

You can find out what it is doing on the following pages.

Thus, the amino acids L-Arginine and L-Citrulline act

L-Arginine is a proteinogenic amino acid. That is, proteins (proteins) are formed therefrom. **We need only 8 essential amino acids** through our diet. That is, 8 amino acids must be fed with the food so that we do not get sick. And then there are **two semi-essential amino acids**. These are, so to

speak, "semi-essential". Normally, we do not need it, but in the case of diseases, stress or sport, the body no longer suffers with the production of these 2 semi-essential amino acids, and they should be fed with the food, resulting in 10 essential amino acids (8 essential amino acids) And 2 semi-essential). L-Arginine is one of these two semi-essential amino acids. Arginine is the only precursor of the neurotransmitter nitric oxide (NO). This nitric oxide controls the expansion of the vessels (the "vascular tone") and thus the blood flow and the blood pressure. **In the absence of L-arginine, this has a detrimental effect on the blood vessels (they narrow), leading to hypertension and ultimately to arteriosclerosis**
(study 4-1).

Much L-Arginine is involved in:

Pumpkin seeds *approx. 5,300 mg*
Peanuts*: approximately 3,500 mg*
Peas*, dried about 2,000 mg*
Pine nuts*: approx. 2.500 mg*
Walnuts*: approximately 2,200 mg*
Soybeans *about 2,200 mg*

Hazelnuts *about 2.000 mg*
Oatmeal: *approx. 800 mg*
All data are in each case based on 100 g.

If you are already suffering from arteriosclerosis, however, it is advisable to take a prescription to increase L-arginine levels. Powder are the most favorable. Tablets are the most expensive. L-arginine is well bio-available with 68% *(4-2)*, which means that it can be used for the body. However, the disadvantage of L-arginine is its very short half-life of 70 min. *(4-2)*. This means that after this time, the arginine is already half-degraded. For this reason, there is an even better amino acid, namely the L-citrulline. This is considered a dwell time prolonger and maintains the arginine level at a stable level as it provides for the time-delayed conversion of citrulline to arginine, which takes place in the liver. **Particularly rich in Citrulline are watermelons**, especially their shells. Now one might think: Why do we still need L-arginine, if L-citrulline is much better because it is converted into L-arginine anyway? According to scientific studies, however, **the combination of L-arginine** and L-citrulline has proved to be much more effective *(study 3)* than when only one of the two is taken. If, however, you want to go the minimalistic way and just want to take one of the two, then you should prefer to use L-Citrullin, in order to delay the time delay. So you always have a constant L-arginine level. Both amino acids are commercially available as over-the-counter food supplements. Already a few grams are sufficient to increase circulation and improve vascular health.

The undefined influence of prostaglandins on the blood flow and the fairytale of the inflammatory omega 6

These are so-called tissue hormones. They were discovered for the first time in the secretion of the prostate. Hence the name prostaglandins. Meanwhile, it is known that prostaglandins are produced in all tissues. Prostaglandins are not produced in a particular organ and then released into the body's circulation, but are produced directly on site. There are 3 basic types of prostaglandins:

Series 1: Preparation is carried out using the omega-6 fatty acid gamma-linolenic acid. The main prostaglandin in this series is the **prostaglandin E1, which is extremely powerful for blood circulation** and dilates the vessels. It strongly inhibits platelet aggregation (clumping together of blood platelets) and therefore prevents the formation of thromboses.

Series 2: Preparation takes place by means of the essential omega-6 fatty acid linoleic acid, as well as by arachidonic acid from animal foodstuffs (e.g., pork loin). The main prostaglandin in this series is the Prostaglandin E2. Similar to the E1, the E2 also has a strong circulation-promoting effect, but probably somewhat weaker than the E1.

Series 3: The effect of the 3 series has so far been poorly researched. According to today's knowledge, it is anti-inflammatory and can only be synthesized by omega-3 fatty acids.

But let's look at the details of what prostaglandin is:

Prostaglandin E1: This is for you the most important prostaglandin to increase the blood flow! It is even used in emergency medicine under the name "Alprostadil" to treat acute circulatory disorders. The vascular endothelial growth factor (VEGF) protein also inhibits thrombocyte aggregation (clumping of blood platelets), it inhibits proliferation (cell proliferation) and increases the cAMP (cyclic adenosine monophosphate) in many tissues. It also activates the T-lymphocytes (the lymphocytes formed in the thymus), prostaglandin E1 also strengthens the immune defense and also the bone resorption (bone structure) is stimulated by the E-prostaglandins *(Study 19)*. It should also be mentioned that prostaglandin E1 is 20 times more potent than prostaglandin E2 *(study 333)* and that the ratio of both prostaglandins is usually shifted unfavorably (too much E2, too little E1). It is currently disputed (status 2017) whether both prostaglandins bind to the same receptors (EP1, EP2, EP3 and EP4). However, due to the present study situation, all this suggests *(study 333)*. This means that both prostaglandins compete for the same receptors!

Prostaglandin E2: Almost as effective as the E1 and, in addition, the prostaglandin E2 protects you from the formation of a neutralizing mucus of the stomach and esophagus *(Study 20)*. If you often have heartburn (reflux), then a prostaglandin E2 deficiency could be the cause. In addition, prostaglandin E2 has very regulating properties on the immune system and also causes a new formation of blood vessels, similar to the prostaglandin E1. Various studies have shown that prostaglandin E2 leads to a marked increase in the blood flow in the kidneys (study 1) and also bone resorption (bone structure) is stimulated by the e-prostaglandins *(study 19)*.

Prostaglandin D2: Promotes sleep, inhibits thrombocyte aggregation (clumping of blood platelets), promotes vasodilatation (enlargement of the blood vessels) in the kidneys, as well as bronchoconstriction (narrowing of the blood vessels in the bronchi, hence also the connection with asthma) and promotes water reabsorption small intestine. Although it is part of the 2-day prostaglandins, scientists have found that the prostaglandin D2 formed from arachidonic acid is anti-inflammatory *(Study 30)*. And the so-called "inflammation-promoting" prostaglandins not only trigger an inflammation but also ensure that these are terminated again. It is therefore not beneficial for the body to block "prostaglandins" stimulating "inflammation-promoting", as is done with the school-medical COX inhibitors.

Prostaglandin I2 (prostacycline): PGI2 together with PGE2 is the main prostaglandin involved in the inflammatory process. But you know now: This only applies if an inflammation has already been present! It increases the vascular permeability (the permeability of blood vessels, which causes the tissue swelling), is involved in the development of the redness and intensifies the pain. Prostacycline is the most powerful thrombocyte aggregation inhibitor and therefore protects against thrombosis like no other prostaglandin! Prostacycline improves and suppresses blood circulation. It is mainly formed in the vascular endothelium and the smooth muscle and has a blood vessel-dilating, cell-proliferation-inhibiting and cell-protective effect.

Prostaglandin F2-alpha: Promotes the contraction of the smooth muscle and is understood as an antagonist (opponent) to the prostaglandin E2.

Thromboxan A2: Can be viewed as an opponent of prostaglandin I2 (prostacycline). It is mainly formed by thrombocytes and promotes platelet aggregation. This is important, so that you do not bleed at injuries (sloppily said). Furthermore, it causes vessel constriction.

What are the criteria for which prostaglandins are formed?

- The consumption of most linoleic acid-containing oils (sunflower oil, thistle oil, grape seed oil) is always the formation of arachidonic acid and then the prostaglandins of the series 2 (and ONLY the series 2)! *(Study 12)*

- If an oil is consumed where the gamma-linolenic acid already exists (borage oil, evening primrose oil, currant seed oil), the prostaglandins of the series 1 are formed therefrom *(study 16)*. However, there are no vegetable oils where only gamma-linolenic acid is present alone. For all oils where gamma-linolenic acid is present also contain extremely high amounts of linoleic acid and this is converted to arachidonic acid. (GLA), **borage oil (20-25% GLA)**, black currant oil (15-20% GLA) and night-candle oil (10% GLA).

- If, in addition to the gamma-linolenic acid (borage oil, evening primrose oil ...), omega-3 fatty acids are also consumed (namely the ready-metabolized EPA and DHA from salmon oil), gamma-linolenic acid becomes even more (so-called anti-inflammatory) prostaglandins Of the series 1. **In one study, the administration of borage oil + salmon oil resulted in 73 nmol / mg of prostaglandin E1 compared to 39.7 nmol / mg when borage oil alone. When administered salmon oil alone, only 29 nmol / mg.** And when the sun flower oil oil alone (rich in omega-6-linoleic acid, but not gamma-linolenic acid such as borage oil) was administered, it was less than 0.1 nmol / mg Prostaglandin E1. *(Study 13).*

Why healthy people through Omega 6 can not get inflammation

After consumption of omega-6 rich food, the arachidonic acid accumulates in cell membranes and is converted from there to the prostaglandins of the series 2 (in particular prostaglandin I2 and E2) if necessary. Prerequisite for the conversion of arachidonic acid to prostaglandins are 2 enzymes:

Cyclooxygenase 1 (COX-1) and

Cyclooxygenase 2 (COX-2)

The difference between these two enzymes is easily explained: COX-1 is found in tissues of the whole body. **COX-2 additionally in inflamed tissue.** While the prostaglandin E2 synthesis via COX-1 performs normal-routine activities for the maintenance of the body functions, such as the formation of neutralizing mucus of the stomach or a blood circulation-promoting effect, only the pathway via COX-2 acts to promote inflammation. Therefore, healthy people can consume much omega-6-rich linoleic acid without getting inflammation therefrom, while in the case of sick people (osteoarthritis, gout, etc.), linoleic acid may lead to more severe disease symptoms. Many people are of the opinion that Omega 6 is basically the cause of its inflammation-induced disease. But from my point of view this is certainly not the case. Because healthy people do not feel any inflammation under a high linoleic diet. These can not arise because the COX-2 enzyme is missing and this is synthesized only in inflamed tissue. The COX-2 is thus not formed by the omega-6-linoleic acid, but was already present there before and was synthesized by inflammation (e.g., a sands) in the tissue. The causes of the inflammation are quite different. Usually in a chronic poisoning (or sunglasses, as an example). If people get pimple after a high consumption of omega-6-rich vegetable oil, then most of the pesticides or oil fried or fried. It is not surprising, of course, that inflammation occurs, because polyunsaturated fatty acids are very unstable. They are very susceptible to oxidation. Grape seed oil should be particularly stressed with pesticides. This even applies to organic oils. The consumer protection institutes reported. In any case, however, BIO oils are preferable to the conventional ones.

To date, the widespread belief that prostaglandins of the series 1 + 3 are anti-inflammatory, while those of the series 2 (from arachidonic acid) have an inflammatory effect. But if you read the scientific publications as well as the numerous experience reports of people who consumed high-dose omega 6, then you can not assume that Omega 6 is inflammatory. Prostaglandins have an immunoregulatory effect. In a study published in 2009, scientists found that prostaglandins of the series 2 (in particular prostaglandin D2 and F2-alpha) also have an anti-inflammatory effect *(study 30)*. However, since inflamed tissue is rich in the enzyme cyclooxigenase-2 (COX-2), prostaglandins are increasingly formed at the inflamed parts of the body. In any case, you should not believe that prostaglandins are the cause of inflammation! For the inflammation must have been there <u>before</u> an excessive prostaglandin production can take place at all. COX-2 is also found in other parts of the body (e.g., in the spinal cord, even if no inflammation is present). But so that inflammation caused by Omega 6 can arise at all, an inflammation must have been there before! And even then it is not that Omega 6 leads to inflammation without end. On the contrary, healing is initiated and this is confirmed by the experience reports. Thus, omega-6 fatty acids can never be the cause of inflammation. This is really brought on by the hair!

The widespread enzyme deficiency

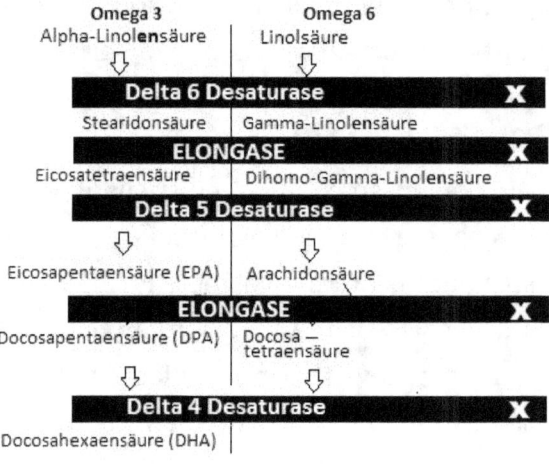

Grafik: © Christian Meyer-Esch

In the diagram above, you will see that a total of 4 different enzymes ensure that the further metabolic intermediates and finally the arachidonic acid or eicosapentaenoic acid (EPA) are formed from the starting substances (linoleic acid / omega 6) or alpha linolenic acid (omega 3) , Which ultimately results in the formation of the prostaglandins. In other words, no prostaglandins are formed at all on the first enzyme, the delta-6-desaturase! Now some will probably have their fun and think "This is wonderful. Then I do not need an aspirin anymore. " But it is not so wonderful. The body is strongly dependent on prostaglandins, as I have already explained in detail in this book.

If the first two enzymes, the delta-6-desaturase and the elongase are active and lack only on the 3rd enzyme (the delta-5-desaturase), this would not be quite so bad. For this, the body could still form the prostaglandins of the series 1 and when fish oil is consumed, also the prostaglandins of the 3rd series. But of course this is not our goal. Because we want all 3 prostaglandin series. So now it's about rebuilding the organism so that all the enzymes work again.

In addition to diabetics who almost always have these enzyme deficiencies *(study 222)*, it is assumed that even people who eat a lot of arachidonic acid through the diet (which therefore consume many animal products) have this enzyme deficiency because the body probably thinks that it is This enzyme no longer needs, since enough "finished" arachidonic acid is consumed. These people have anything but a prostaglandin 2 deficiency. They are likely to have more than enough. What is missing in these people are the prostaglandins of the series 1. Because these can only be formed by means of vegetable omega 6 oils, in particular borageschöl, Nachtkerzenöl and the oil of the black currant. Usually together with fish oil. In the case of the sole consumption of fish (oil) + arachidonic acid from meat, however, prostaglandin 1 production does not occur.

And so you revive the enzyme activity of the delta-6-desaturase (study 222):

- By moderate diet (increases enzyme activity by 300%)
- By avoiding diabetes
- Vitamin B3
- Vitamin B6
- zinc
- vitamin C
- Melatonin (The "sleep hormone")

Beware of acetylsalicylic acid and other COX inhibitors

The use of so-called COX-inhibitors can only be warned. It inhibits the enzymes needed for prostaglandin production. And thus, by taking these drugs comes a prostaglandin deficiency. Although there are now also COX inhibitors, which selectively inhibit COX-2 only. However, studies have shown that this leads to more arachidonic acid remaining for COX-1, which then leads to more thromboxane A2, which increases blood coagulation. Although this can partially compensate with Omega 3. But healthy COX inhibitors are not in any case healthy. They now know the importance of the prostaglandins in the body. When inflammation occurs in the body, this has very different causes (usually too much uric acid and / or toxins). But not too much at Omega 6 or Prostaglandins. An inhibition of this is therefore only short-term symptom suppression and aggravates the health situation still further. *(Study 66a)*

What causes the chronic inflammation of the arteries?

- **Lipidperoxidation**

- **Diabetes** (Chronically elevated blood glucose values)

- **Increased blood pressure (Hypertonie)**

In response to one of the above causes, the body reacts with inflammation, providing cholesterol and limescale deposits to "patch" the blood vessels damaged by inflammation. In the short term this is a good thing. In the long term, however, this leads to more and more damaged blood vessels. These get more and more deposits over time, until they eventually close completely. This can then lead to myocardial infarction, stroke, and / or to a peripheral arterial blood circulation disorder.

But let us examine in detail what the actual causes are and how to avoid them:

Lipidperoxidation:

This is the oxidation of fatty acids. If you consume a fat or oil, which is strongly heated (by frying or frying), so-called "free radicals" arise. These are wild oxygen molecules that are missing an electron. And in search of the missing electron, they steal it from other substances in the blood. Thus, a whole chain reaction is triggered, which can only be stopped by antioxidants. If you consume an oil that has not been heated, they usually do not have this problem. Unless the oil is very old or has been exposed to air for a long time. The heating of fat is one of the biggest problems of modern man. No animal would ever get the idea and get fat. Fats are very reactive and unstable. And the more unsaturated fatty acids it contains, the more susceptible to oxidation is it. But the unsaturated fatty acids are so important to us. We need only two essential fatty acids: linoleic acid (omega 6) and alpha-linolenic acid (omega 3). All other fatty acids are not essential! It can make the body itself. Here is a brief overview, where the essential (ie vital) fatty acids occur everywhere (the list is not complete!)

Linoleic Acid (Omega 6):

Grape seed oil	approx. 65%
Safflower oil (safflower oil)	approx. 65%
Hemp oil	approx. 50%
Soybean oil	approx. 55%
Cotton seed oil	approx. 50%
Wheat germ oil	approx. 50%
Maize germ oil	approx. 50%
Sunflower oil	approx. 60%
Sunflower oil for frying	approx. 5%
Rapeseed oil	approx. 25%
Linseed oil	approx. 15%
Olive oil	approx. 5%
Walnuts	approx 34%
Peanuts	approx 14%
Hazelnuts	approx. 8%

Alpha-linolenic acid (Omega 3):

Linseed oil:	approx. 60%
Chiael:	approx 60%
Perilla oil:	approx 60%
Sacha Inchi Oil:	approx. 50%
Leindotter oil:	approx. 35%
Hemp oil:	approx. 15%
Walnut oil:	approx. 13%
Rape oil:	approx. 9%
Soybean oil:	approx. 8%

If you want to learn more about the topic of "essential fatty acids" and the effects of those on health, then I recommend you my book

„The Omega 6 Fallacy: POPULATION DEFICIENT instead of inflammatory mediator" www.insider-remedies.com

No oil is therefore suitable for frying since all fats are unstable. The most harmless is, however, the coconut fat, since it contains the least unsaturated fatty acids. The best thing, however, would be to boil only with water or not   at   all. So if you consume an oxidized fat (which has been exposed to air or heated for a long time), a firework of free radicals is created in your blood vessels. And in response to these chronic inflammatory conditions, the body reacts with lime and cholesterol deposits. But also with hardened connective tissue, which ultimately makes the blood vessels bulky and porous and makes them more and more narrow with the years. Lipid peroxidation is therefore one of the causes of calcified blood vessels and this is also scientifically proven *(Study   27)*.
The good news is: We are not without

protection! Besides the avoiding of oxidized fat there is also a "Detox". These are fat-soluble antioxidants, in particular vitamin E, alpha lipoic acid and chlorella seaweed.

Do the self-test:

„Malondialdehyd" Is a free radical test for the urine. I have already done many tests of this kind and can say from experience: Whenever I ate fries, the value 1-2 hours afterwards was significantly increased! However, I have taken vitamin E, chlorella seaweed or alpha-linolenic acid to me before the fries consumption, an increased value! The strongest effect was the alpha-lipoic acid (a high-concentration body-borne antioxidant). With his help I had zero free radicals in the urine despite fries consumption! Chlorella seaweed also produced a similar result in a dose-dependent manner. Vitamin E was not quite as effective, but also effective.

Diabetes:

What now has the dozens of diabetes with arteriosclerosis to do, ask yourself. This is actually quite easy to answer: If the blood glucose is no longer or insufficiently degraded as in diabetes, this leads to inflammation in the blood vessels, whereupon the body then reacts with the storage of cholesterol and lime in the vessels *(Studies 75, 76)* , For healthy blood vessels it is therefore of particular importance not to have diabetes.

Increased blood pressure:

Various studies have shown that elevated blood pressure can damage the vessels and lead to atherosclerosis *(Studies 77, 78, 79)*. This is also logical because you must remember that a permanently increased pressure in the vessels damages them. Imagine a garden hose, where the water always comes out with very high pressure. Such garden hoses are, of course, worn more quickly than those where the water comes out with normal pressure. But, conversely, deposits in the vessels cause the blood pressure to increase. The question is: What was first? The high blood pressure or arteriosclerosis? In principle, it does not matter. **Ensure optimal blood pressure of 120/80 (systolic / diastolic)** through the insider healing procedures described in this book so that your blood vessels remain healthy. Very important for optimal blood pressure is the deficiency mineral potassium. Ideally with simultaneously reduced salt consumption.

C-Reactive Protein: The most important blood parameter

No other blood value for heart attack and stroke risk is more relevant and more important than the C-reactive protein. Why is that? Many ways can lead to occluded blood vessels such as diabetes, deficiency of magnesium, lack of prostaglandins or amino acids, etc. One thing all these causes have in common: It is always an inflammation that takes place in the blood vessels! A marker in the blood for such inflammation is the C-reactive protein, a protein that is formed in the liver. However, the "normal" C-reactive protein is more "hs C-reactive protein". HS stands for highly sensitive. Thus, very small concentrations can be measured by sensitive measuring methods. In studies, it has been shown clearly that the C-reactive protein is a potent risk factor for atherosclerosis and the resulting diseases *(studies 72, 73, 74)*. As reported by the "German Ärzteblatt", **the patients with an acute vascular closure died with 3.2 µg / ml the highest CRP blood levels.** (German Ärzteblatt 2002, 99 (17): A-1132 / B-942 / C-886).

Normal value hsCrP:

Under 0,1 mg/dl

The out-of-control potassium-sodium ratio

Surely you have heard a lot about the so-called "over-acidification". However, there is no over-acidification of the blood. For the PH value of the blood is always kept between PH 7.35 and 7.45 by means of specific regulation mechanisms. So always slightly basic. Thus, only cells and tissues can leach. And here the minerals calcium, magnesium, potassium and sodium play an important role. The minerals deacidify calcium and sodium extracellularly (= outside cells), whereas potassium and magnesium deacidify intracellularly (within the cells). There is no need to worry about a sufficient supply of sodium, because our food is now heavily salted (sodium chloride) so that a lack of sodium is not to be expected. Calcium also takes people too much. Most people are sick through calcification (much too much calcium, at the same time frightening little magnesium). According to the most recent studies, 70% of all people are under-treated with potassium and a **potassium deficiency leads to hypertension! And this in turn causes inflammation in the blood vessels and arteriosclerosis!** People used to eat very much potassium-containing fruit and grain. Sodium, on the other hand, ("The White Gold") was scarce. Today it is exactly the opposite. Sodium is ubiquitous and potassium deficiencyware! In this case, potassium is extremely important, because without sufficient potassium, our cells become acidic! Potassium deficiency can also trigger or promote cancer. There are studies that show a clear correlation. More in my book *"Insider-cures against cancer"*. The recommended daily intake of potassium is 4.7 g per day, but hardly any human being. But let us take a look at how much potassium intake was in the past:

Earlier:	Today:
Potassium 10 g / day	Potassium 3,5 g / day
Sodium 0,8 g / day	Sodium 4,3 g / day

(source: WHO **1054**)

So you see: the ratio of potassium to sodium was earlier at 10: 1. Today it is in the best case at 1: 1, whereby even more sodium than potassium is consumed. Potassium and sodium are opposites. And the more sodium we take to us (and this is a lot nowadays, for salt is almost everywhere), the more potassium we need.

Warning: Do not exceed 10 g per day! If you have kidney failure, consult your doctor. Excessive doses can lead to heart failure.

How do myocardial infarction and stroke develop?

In a heart attack, a blood clot closes one of the coronary arteries. The blood flow in the vessel is interrupted by its occlusion. If the blood supply is not restored within a short time, some of the heart muscle tissue dies. The same happens in a stroke, only in the brain. In addition, in about 15% of all strokes, there is still the hemorrhagic stroke, where it leads to a hemorrhage into the brain instead of a vascular occlusion. It can also be that a blood clot forms in the heart, which then migrates into the brain (or vice versa) and the blood circulation in the brain is then blocked. This is the case in 85% of all strokes and is called ischemic stroke. The cause is the same with all: broken, inflamed blood vessels, thus arteriosclerosis. The signs of a heart attack are sudden, violent pain in the chest, which can radiate into the left arm, belly, back, or teeth. Also a feeling of tightness in the chest, nausea and shortness of breath. Typical signs of a stroke are half-sided paralysis, numbness, speech impairment, visual impairment, or facial disability.

Thick Blood: Risk Factor for Heart Attack and Stroke

The more viscid the blood, the more the heart must work to pump the blood through the body. Thick blood flows slower and increases the risk of thrombosis, myocardial infarction and   stroke. By means of the blood parameter hematocrit, it is possible to determine how thick or thin the blood is. This is often found in the laboratory, since it is one of the standard blood tests, which are paid by the statutory health insurance funds. For the patient, thorough blood is taken from the vein, the specimen is treated with a anticoagulant and centrifuged in a tube. The solid constituents are used

- **Erythrocytes**
  (Red blood cells, used for oxygen supply)
- **Leukocytes**
  (White blood cells, defense cells of the immune system)
- **Platelets**
  (Blood clotting)

Clearly visible from the blood plasma. Women usually have thinner blood than men, possibly due to menstrual bleeding. Accordingly, the norm values for men and women also differ:

Standard value of hematocrit:
Men 36 - 48%
Women 35 - 45%

A suitable means to lower the hematocrit is much to drink. In one, it was shown that the intake of omega-3 fatty acids (fish oil, 1-2 g / day) significantly increased the effect of anticoagulant warfarin (a drug which inhibits blood coagulation). **The INR value rose by Omega 3 from 2.8 to 4.3.** *(Study 80)*. Omega-3 fatty acids are therefore a suitable means to dilute the blood. They have no influence on hematocrit! For vegans, this should also be possible using vegetable omega 3 made from linseed oil. Note, however, that the blood must not become too thin. Follow the recommended standard values and discuss high-quality omega-3 fatty acids with your doctor. Especially if you already take a blood thinning drug such as warfarin.

Uric Acid: A Risk for Arteriosclerosis?

A study from 2007 showed that uric acid is not associated with coronary arteriosclerosis. Any correlation reported in other studies was probably due to the relationship between high serum uric acid levels and other cardiovascular risk factors *(study 70)*.

The insider cures at a glance

Die Insider-cures against...

Vessels Calcification:
Vitamin K2, Magnesium, Inositol,
Vitamin D (The right amount!) and Lysine.

Lipoprotein A:
Vitamin C, Lysine, Niacin (Vitamin B3) and
L-Carnitine

Triglycerides:
Niacin (Vitamin B3) from 500 mg, Omega-3-
fatty acids, L-Carnitin, Lecithin

Cholesterol:
Niacin (Vitamin B3), Lecithin

Homocysteine:
Vitamin B6, Vitamin B9 (Folic acid), Vitamin
B12 and Lecithin

Fibrin:
Serrapeptase

Fibrosis:
Milk thistle, Taurine, Niacin

Lipidperoxidation:
Alpha-lipoic acid, Vitamin E, Chlorella-seaweed, Vitamin A, Beta Carotine

Stiff, inelastic blood vessels:
Silicea, Omega 3-fatty acids and the treatments against calcification.

General circulatory disorders:
Prostaglandin E1 (self-production by means of borage oil) and the amino acids L-arginine and L-citrulline

High blood pressure:
Potassium (10 g per day)
(Except for dialysis patients or people with renal insufficiency)

Relevant blood values at a glance

The most important values are marked in bold

Parameter:	setpoint:
Total cholesterol (page 35)	to 200 mg/dl
HDL-Cholesterol (page 35)	Mindestens 45 mg/dl
LDL-Cholesterol (page 35)	to 130 mg/dl
Triglyceride (page 44)	under 200 mg/dl
Lipoprotein A (page 27)	**under 30 mg/dl**
Homocysteine (page 46)	**under 5 mcmol/l**
Fibrinogen (page 53)	1,8 - 3,5 g/l
Magnesium (page 13)	0,8 - 1,1 mmol/l.
HbA1c (only for patients with Diabetes)	under 5,7%
Free Radicals (Malondialdehyd) (page 93)	Urine test
Blood pressure (page 95)	**to 120 / 80** (systolic / diastolic)
Hämatocrit (page 101)	Men 36 – 48%, Women 35 – 45%

Hs C-reactive Protein (hs-CrP) (page 96)	Under 0,1 mg/dl
Vitamin D (page 20)	35-60 ng/ml

List of studies and sources

(1) Prostaglandin E2 induzierte Veränderungen in der renalen Blutfluss, renalen interstitiellen hydrostatischen Druck und Natrium-Ausscheidung in der Ratte.

https://www.ncbi.nlm.nih.gov/pubmed/2093936

(2) Normwerte von Homocystein:

http://www.homocystein-netzwerk.de/homocystein/homocystein-werte-deuten/

(3) Die orale Supplementierung mit einer Kombination von L-Citrullin und L-Arginin erhöht die Plasma-L-Argininkonzentration schnell und verbessert die NO-Bioverfügbarkeit

https://www.ncbi.nlm.nih.gov/pubmed/25445598

(4) Orale L-Arginin-Supplementierung bei Patienten mit milder arterieller Hypertonie und ihre Wirkung auf den Plasmaspiegel von asymmetrischem Dimethylarginin, L-Citrulin, L-Arginin und Antioxidansstatus (Arginin erhöht auch den Citrulin-Spiegel)

https://www.ncbi.nlm.nih.gov/pubmed/23161038

(4-1) L-Arginin bei koronarer Atherosklerose.

https://www.ncbi.nlm.nih.gov/pubmed/11077122

(4-2) L-Arginin Halbwertszeit und Bioverfügbarkeit

http://naturaldatabase.therapeuticresearch.com/nd/PrintVersion.aspx?id=875&AspxAutoDetectCookieSupport=1

(5) SYNTHESE VON INOSITOL BEI MÄUSEN

https://www.ncbi.nlm.nih.gov/pmc/articles/PMC2135247/

(6) Arteriosklerose- chronischer Entzündungszustand

https://www.ncbi.nlm.nih.gov/pubmed/11001066

(7) Atherosklerose und Omega-3-Fettsäuren in den Populationen eines Fischerdorfes und eines Bauerndorfes in Japan.

https://www.ncbi.nlm.nih.gov/pubmed/11164437

(8) Ernährung hat keinen Einfluss auf Cholesterinspiegel:

https://www.ncbi.nlm.nih.gov/pubmed/11111098

(9) Verlust der Delta-6-Desaturase-Aktivität als Schlüsselfaktor für die Alterung.

https://www.ncbi.nlm.nih.gov/pubmed/6270521

(10) Autoimmunität und Prostaglandine

https://www.ncbi.nlm.nih.gov/pubmed/7035343

(11) Dualer Einfluss von Alterung und Vitamin B6-Mangel auf die Delta-6-Desaturierung

https://www.ncbi.nlm.nih.gov/pubmed/10189072

(12) Die Auswirkungen von Nachtkerzenöl, Safloröl und Paraffin auf die Plasmafettsäuren im Menschen: Wahl eines geeigneten Placebo für klinische Studien an Primelöl.

https://www.ncbi.nlm.nih.gov/pubmed/1871175

(13) Maus-Peritoneal-Makrophagen-Prostaglandin-E1-Synthese wird durch diätetische Gamma-Linolensäure verändert.

https://www.ncbi.nlm.nih.gov/pubmed/1322453

(14) Indices der Fettsäure-Desaturase-Aktivität bei gesunden menschlichen Probanden: Auswirkungen verschiedener Arten von Nahrungsfett

https://www.ncbi.nlm.nih.gov/pubmed/23414551

(15) Mögliche Rolle von Prostaglandin E1 bei affektiven Störungen und beim Alkoholismus

https://www.ncbi.nlm.nih.gov/pmc/articles/PMC1601822/

(16) Bedeutung der Nahrungs-Gamma-Linolensäure in der menschlichen Gesundheit und Ernährung.

https://www.ncbi.nlm.nih.gov/pubmed/9732298

(17) Gamma-Linolensäure in Borretschöl kehrt die epidermale Hyperproliferation bei Meerschweinchen um

https://www.ncbi.nlm.nih.gov/pubmed/12368400

(18) Die Co-Supplementierung von gesunden Frauen mit Fischöl und Nachtkerzenöl erhöht die Plasma-Docosahexaensäure, die Gamma-Linolensäure und die Dihomo-Gamma-Linolensäure-Konzentrationen, ohne die Arachidonsäure-Konzentrationen zu reduzieren.

https://www.ncbi.nlm.nih.gov/pubmed/17678567

(18a) Wirkung von Rizinusöl-Diät auf die Synthese von Prostaglandin E2 bei schwangeren Ratten

https://www.ncbi.nlm.nih.gov/pubmed/11263183

(19) Relation between progression and regression of atherosclerotic left main coronary artery disease and serum cholesterol levels as assessed with serial long-term (> or =12 months) follow-up intravascular ultrasound.

https://www.ncbi.nlm.nih.gov/pubmed/14623804

(20) Optimal low-density lipoprotein is 50 to 70 mg/dl: lower is better and physiologically normal.

https://www.ncbi.nlm.nih.gov/pubmed/15172426

(21) Die Wirkung von Granatapfel-Extrakt auf koronare Arterien-Atherosklerose in SR-BI / APOE Doppel-Knockout-Mäusen.

https://www.ncbi.nlm.nih.gov/pubmed/23528829

(22) Granatapfelsaft Verbrauch für 3 Jahre von Patienten mit Carotis-Stenose reduziert die gemeinsame Karotis Intima-Media Dicke, Blutdruck und LDL-Oxidation.

https://www.ncbi.nlm.nih.gov/pubmed/15158307

(23) Granatapfelsaft Supplementierung zu atherosklerotischen Mäusen reduziert Makrophagen Lipidperoxidation, zelluläre Cholesterin-Akkumulation und Entwicklung der Atherosklerose.

https://www.ncbi.nlm.nih.gov/pubmed/11481398

(24) Granatapfelsaft Verbrauch hemmt Serum-Angiotensin-Converting-Enzym-Aktivität und reduziert den systolischen Blutdruck.

https://www.ncbi.nlm.nih.gov/pubmed/11500191

(25) Unterschiedliche Beziehungen zu frühen Atherosclerosis zwischen Vitamin C aus Supplements gegen Lebensmittel in der Los Angeles Atherosclerosis Study

https://www.ncbi.nlm.nih.gov/pmc/articles/PMC3447163

(26) Liponsäure-Effekte auf etablierte Atherosklerose

https://www.ncbi.nlm.nih.gov/pmc/articles/PMC3075920/

(27) Lipidoxidationsprodukte haben entgegengesetzte Effekte auf die Verkalkung der vaskulären Zellen- und Knochenzelldifferenzierung. Eine mögliche Erklärung für das Paradoxon der arteriellen Verkalkung bei osteoporotischen Patienten.

https://www.ncbi.nlm.nih.gov/pubmed/9108780

(34) Die kardiovaskulären Effekte von Leinsamen und seine Omega-3-Fettsäure, alpha-Linolensäure

https://www.ncbi.nlm.nih.gov/pmc/articles/PMC2989356/

(28) Leinsamenöl und Fischöl Kapselverbrauch verändert menschliche rote Blutkörperchen n-3-Fettsäure-Zusammensetzung: eine Mehrfachdosierung Vergleich von 2 Quellen von n-3-Fettsäure.

https://www.ncbi.nlm.nih.gov/pubmed/18779299

(29) Diätetische Substitution mit einem alpha-Linolensäure-reichen Pflanzenöl erhöht die Eicosapentaensäure-Konzentrationen im Gewebe.

https://www.ncbi.nlm.nih.gov/pubmed/7910999?dopt=Abstract

(719) Leinsamenöl erhöht die Plasmakonzentrationen von kardioprotektiven (n-3) Fettsäuren beim Menschen.

https://www.ncbi.nlm.nih.gov/pubmed/16365063

(30) Die entzündungshemmenden Wirkungen von Prostaglandinen

https://www.ncbi.nlm.nih.gov/pubmed/19240648

(31) Eine Erhöhung der Triglyceride, die eine verminderte Triglycerid-Clearance widerspiegelt, ist möglicherweise nicht pathogen - relevant für hochkohlehydrathaltige Diäten

https://www.ncbi.nlm.nih.gov/pubmed/15504577

(31-2) Triglyceride und Herz-Kreislauf-Risiko

https://www.ncbi.nlm.nih.gov/pmc/articles/PMC2822144/

(31-3) Wirkmechanismus von Niacin

https://www.ncbi.nlm.nih.gov/pubmed/18375237

(32) Niedriges Serumsex-Hormon-bindendes Globulin: Marker der Entzündung?

https://www.ncbi.nlm.nih.gov/pubmed/22293276

(33) Testosteron, SHBG und differentielle weiße Blutkörperchen in mittleren und älteren Männern.

https://www.ncbi.nlm.nih.gov/pubmed/22221653

(35) Diätetisches L-Lysin verhindert die arterielle Verkalkung bei Adenin-induzierten urämischen Ratten.

https://www.ncbi.nlm.nih.gov/pubmed/24652795

(36) Verkalkung von Perikardgewebe vorbehandelt mit verschiedenen Aminosäuren.

https://www.ncbi.nlm.nih.gov/pubmed/8652775

(37) Diätetische L-Lysin und Calcium-Stoffwechsel beim Menschen.

https://www.ncbi.nlm.nih.gov/pubmed/1486246

(38) Fibrinogen-, Fibrin- und Fibrinabbauprodukte in Bezug auf Arteriosklerose.

https://www.ncbi.nlm.nih.gov/pubmed/3524931

(39) Fibrinogen und Atherosklerose

https://www.ncbi.nlm.nih.gov/pubmed/8379153

(40) Wirkung von Vitamin C auf die Endothelfunktion bei Gesundheit und Krankheit: eine systematische Überprüfung und Metaanalyse von randomisierten kontrollierten Studien

https://www.ncbi.nlm.nih.gov/pubmed/24792921

(41) Vitamin C aus NEMs erhöht die Arteriosklerose:

https://www.ncbi.nlm.nih.gov/pmc/articles/PMC34471
63/

(42) Atherofibrose - ein einzigartiger und gemeinsamer Prozess der Krankheit Pathogenese der Atherosklerose und Fibrose - Lektionen für die Entwicklung von Biomarkern

https://www.ncbi.nlm.nih.gov/pmc/articles/PMC35604
83/

(42-2) Perifollikuläre Fibrose: pathogenetische Rolle bei der androgenetischen Alopezie.

https://www.ncbi.nlm.nih.gov/pubmed/16755026

(42-3) Muster der Myokardfibrose

https://www.ncbi.nlm.nih.gov/pubmed/2534137

(42-4) Anti-inflammatory/anti-fibrotic effects of the hepatoprotective silymarin and the schistosomicide praziquantel against Schistosoma mansoni-induced liver fibrosis.

https://www.ncbi.nlm.nih.gov/pubmed/22236605

(42-5) Niacin dämpft die Bomycin-induzierte Lungenfibrose im Hamster.

https://www.ncbi.nlm.nih.gov/pubmed/1698227

(42-6) Regression of liver fibrosis by taurine in rats fed alcohol: effects on collagen accumulation, selected cytokines and stellate cell activation.

https://www.ncbi.nlm.nih.gov/pubmed/20813107

(43) Androgen-induzierte Progression der arteriellen Verkalkung in Apolipoprotein E-Null-Mäusen ist von Plaque-Wachstum und Lipid-Ebenen abgekoppelt.

https://www.ncbi.nlm.nih.gov/pubmed/19176322

(44) Entzündung und vaskuläre Verkalkung

https://www.ncbi.nlm.nih.gov/pubmed/15627739

(45) Verkalkungen, arterielle Steifheit und Atherosklerose

https://www.ncbi.nlm.nih.gov/pubmed/17075212

(46) Magnesium-Aufnahme ist umgekehrt mit Koronararterienverkalkung assoziiert: die Framingham Herzstudie

https://www.ncbi.nlm.nih.gov/pubmed/24290571

(47) Weichgewebeverkalkung mit lokaler und oraler Magnesiumtherapie behandelt.

https://www.ncbi.nlm.nih.gov/pubmed/2133625

(48) Untersuchung der Magnesium-Bioverfügbarkeit aus zehn organischen und anorganischen Mg-Salzen bei Mg-abgereicherten Ratten unter Verwendung eines stabilen Isotopenansatzes

https://www.ncbi.nlm.nih.gov/pubmed/16548135

(49) Bioverfügbarkeit von US-kommerziellen Magnesiumpräparaten.

https://www.ncbi.nlm.nih.gov/pubmed/11794633

(50) Magnesium Bioverfügbarkeit aus Mineralwasser. Eine Studie bei erwachsenen Männern

https://www.ncbi.nlm.nih.gov/pubmed/12001016

(51) Mg Citrat fand mehr bioverfügbar als andere Mg-Präparate in einer randomisierten, doppelblinden Studie.

https://www.ncbi.nlm.nih.gov/pubmed/14596323

(52) Magnesium-Bioverfügbarkeit aus Magnesiumcitrat und Magnesiumoxid.

https://www.ncbi.nlm.nih.gov/pubmed/2407766

(53) Lipoprotein (a): medizinische Behandlungsmöglichkeiten für ein schwer fassbares Molekül.

https://www.ncbi.nlm.nih.gov/pubmed/21476974

(54) Vitamin-C-Mangel verursacht Atherosklerose durch die Ablagerung von Lipoprotein(a) in der Gefäßwand von transgenen Mäusen

http://www4ger.dr-rath-foundation.org/DIE_FOUNDATION/LP_a_-Studie_MR_2015Jun18.pdf

(55) Impact of L-carnitine on plasma lipoprotein(a) concentrations: A systematic review and meta-analysis of randomized controlled trials

https://www.ncbi.nlm.nih.gov/pmc/articles/PMC4709689/

(56) The effect of L-carnitine on plasma lipoprotein(a) levels in hypercholesterolemic patients with type 2 diabetes mellitus.

https://www.ncbi.nlm.nih.gov/pubmed/12867219

(57) Inositol und Pantothensäure:

https://www.ncbi.nlm.nih.gov/pmc/articles/PMC2135247/

(58) Phytat (Myo-Inositol-Hexakisphosphat) hemmt kardiovaskuläre Verkalkungen bei Ratten

https://www.ncbi.nlm.nih.gov/pubmed/16146720

(59) Diätetisches Myo-Inositol-Hexaphosphat verhindert dystrophische Verkalkungen in Weichgeweben: eine Pilotstudie bei Wistar-Ratten.

https://www.ncbi.nlm.nih.gov/pubmed/15102518

(60) Phytat reduziert altersbedingte Herz-Kreislauf-Verkalkung.

https://www.ncbi.nlm.nih.gov/pubmed/18508720

(61) Studie einer Myo-Inositol-Hexaphosphat-basierten Creme zur Vermeidung von dystrophischen Calcinose cutis.

https://www.ncbi.nlm.nih.gov/pubmed/15888163

(62) Diätetisches I- Lysin verhindert arterielle Verkalkung bei Adenin-induzierten Uremic-Ratten

https://www.ncbi.nlm.nih.gov/pmc/articles/PMC4147981/

(63) Vitamin D Toxizität bei Erwachsenen: Eine Fallreihe aus einem Bereich mit endemischer Hypovitaminose D:

https://www.ncbi.nlm.nih.gov/pmc/articles/PMC3191699/

(64) Einnahme und Quellen von Phylloquinon (Vitamin K (1) bei 4-jährigen britischen Kindern: Vergleich zwischen 1950 und den 1990er Jahren.

https://www.ncbi.nlm.nih.gov/pubmed/15877910

(65) Verbände der diätetischen Kalziumzufuhr und Kalziumergänzung mit Myokardinfarkt und Schlaganfallrisiko und Gesamt-Herz-Kreislauf-Mortalität in der Heidelberger Kohorte der Europäischen Studieninteresses zur Krebs- und Ernährungsstudie (EPIC-Heidelberg).

https://www.ncbi.nlm.nih.gov/pubmed/22626900

(66) Regression der Warfarin-induzierten medialen Elastocalcinose durch hohe Aufnahme von Vitamin K bei Ratten

https://www.ncbi.nlm.nih.gov/pubmed/17138823

(67) Niacin und Cholesterin: Rolle bei Herz-Kreislauf-Erkrankungen (Review).

https://www.ncbi.nlm.nih.gov/pubmed/12873710

(68) Niacin-Therapie, HDL-Cholesterin und Herz-Kreislauf-Erkrankung: Ist die HDL-Hypothese defekt?

https://www.ncbi.nlm.nih.gov/pmc/articles/PMC4829575/

(69) Homocystein-Ebene und koronare Herzkrankheit Inzidenz: eine systematische Überprüfung und Meta-Analyse.

https://www.ncbi.nlm.nih.gov/pubmed/18990318

(70) Uric acid: a risk factor for coronary atherosclerosis?

https://www.ncbi.nlm.nih.gov/pubmed/17392990

(71) A multi-centre, double-blind study of serrapeptase versus placebo in post-antrotomy buccal swelling

https://www.ncbi.nlm.nih.gov/pubmed/6366808

(72) The connection between C-reactive protein and atherosclerosis

https://www.ncbi.nlm.nih.gov/pubmed/18293141

(73) Inflammation and atherosclerosis: role of C-reactive protein in risk assessment

https://www.ncbi.nlm.nih.gov/pubmed/15050187

(74) Inflammation and atherosclerosis: the value of the high-sensitivity C-reactive protein assay as a risk marker.

https://www.ncbi.nlm.nih.gov/pubmed/11993695

(75) Pathogenesis of atherosclerosis in diabetes and hypertension.

https://www.ncbi.nlm.nih.gov/pubmed/10052643

(76) Atherosclerosis in diabetes mellitus: role of inflammation

https://www.ncbi.nlm.nih.gov/pubmed/17478962

(77) Role of hypertension in atherosclerosis and cardiovascular disease.

https://www.ncbi.nlm.nih.gov/pubmed/136891

(78) Atherosclerosis and hypertension: mechanisms and interrelationships.

https://www.ncbi.nlm.nih.gov/pubmed/1694933

(79) Atherosclerosis and arterial blood pressure in mice.

https://www.ncbi.nlm.nih.gov/pubmed/18045096

(80) Fish oil interaction with warfarin

https://www.ncbi.nlm.nih.gov/pubmed/14742793

(222) Verlust der Delta-6-Desaturase-Aktivität als Schlüsselfaktor für die Alterung.

https://www.ncbi.nlm.nih.gov/pubmed/6270521

(333) Mehrere Rollen von Dihomo-?-Linolensäure gegen Proliferationserkrankungen

https://www.ncbi.nlm.nih.gov/pmc/articles/PMC3295719/

(610) Autoimmunität und Prostaglandine

https://www.ncbi.nlm.nih.gov/pubmed/7035343

(612) Die Auswirkungen von Nachtkerzenöl, Safloröl und Paraffin auf die Plasmafettsäuren im Menschen: Wahl eines geeigneten Placebo für klinische Studien an Primelöl.

https://www.ncbi.nlm.nih.gov/pubmed/1871175

(613) Maus-Peritoneal-Makrophagen-Prostaglandin-E1-Synthese wird durch diätetische Gamma-Linolensäure verändert.

https://www.ncbi.nlm.nih.gov/pubmed/1322453

(616) Bedeutung der Nahrungs-Gamma-Linolensäure in der menschlichen Gesundheit und Ernährung.

https://www.ncbi.nlm.nih.gov/pubmed/9732298

(618) Die Co-Supplementierung von gesunden Frauen mit Fischöl und Nachtkerzenöl erhöht die Plasma-Docosahexaensäure, die Gamma-Linolensäure und die Dihomo-Gamma-Linolensäure-Konzentrationen, ohne die Arachidonsäure-Konzentrationen zu reduzieren.

https://www.ncbi.nlm.nih.gov/pubmed/17678567

(619) Prostaglandin E stimuliert die Knochenbildung

https://www.ncbi.nlm.nih.gov/pmc/articles/PMC2266676/

(620) Prostaglandin EP Rezeptoren und ihre Rollen in Schleimhautschutz und Geschwür Heilung im Magen-Darm-Trakt.

https://www.ncbi.nlm.nih.gov/pubmed/20857620

(630) Die entzündungshemmenden Wirkungen von Prostaglandinen

https://www.ncbi.nlm.nih.gov/pubmed/19240648

Vitamin C vs. Orangensaft:

(855) https://www.ncbi.nlm.nih.gov/pubmed/17349075

(954) Die Auswirkungen von Niacin auf die Lipoprotein-Subklassenverteilung.

https://www.ncbi.nlm.nih.gov/pubmed/15539965

(1054) Natrium/Kalium-Ungleichgewicht
(Weltgesundheitsorganisation):

http://www.who.int/dietphysicalactivity/Elliot-brown-2007.pdf

Photo Credits

Imprint

Editor: Amazon Media EU S.à r.l.,5 Rue Plaetis, L-2338, Luxembourg
Author: Christian Meyer-Esch,
Hoisdorfer Landstr. 97a, 22927 Großhansdorf

About the author:
Christian Meyer-Esch has been working intensively on alternative and holistic medicine for 13 years. He is looking for scientific studies and experience reports worldwide to find solutions, especially for difficult-to-treat diseases. His primary focus is on root causes.